P

Printed in the United States of America
Published by WingSpan Press, Livermore, CA
www.wingspanpress.com
The WingSpan name, logo and colophon
are the trademarks of WingSpan Publishing.

First Edition 2010

ISBN 978-1-59594-428-3
Library of Congress Control Number:
2010941205

p

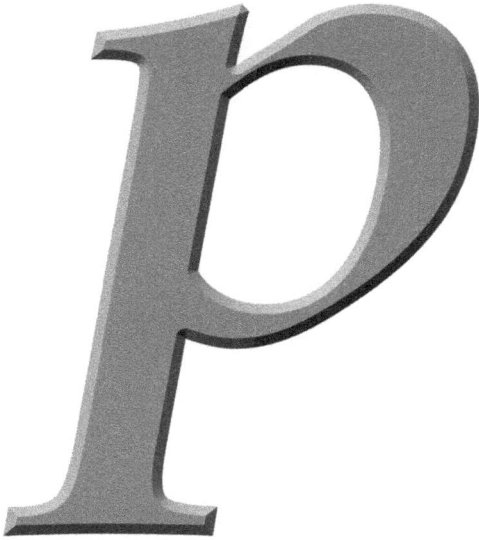

Managing the urinary issues
of prostate cancer surgery

Ed St.Martin

To all the men who find a need
to read this book.
I wish you success in your journey
through cancer surgery and beyond.

And to the friends and family
surrounding you
and helping you on your path.

First, let me explain the title of this book:

$$p$$

You might think it stands for "*p*rostate".
However it needs no interpretation. It
simply stands for "*p*". Or, more descriptively,
*p*ee. Urine, *p*iss, golden showers, or
whatever else you want to call it, it's all the
same. Were it not for my decreased ability
to *p*ee at a relatively young age, I may never
have been diagnosed with *p*rostate cancer
until *p*erhaps it was too late. So, I will
forever be grateful for not being able to *p*ee
well all those years ago.
And for *p*aying attention!

This book however, is more about the *p*eeing
after surgery. I call it the "dirty little secret"
of having *p*rostate cancer surgery — a
radical *p*rostatectomy. You see, most of the
attention during this procedure is *p*laced
on eradication of the cancer. And rightly

so! There's also a *p*lethora of drugs, devices and *p*rocedures available in case you have difficulty with erections following surgery. When it comes to the urinary issues or side effects however, *p*recious little is ever discussed.

But before I delve into the time frame of *p*ost-surgery, let me just say that if you have any difficulty *p*eeing at any age, go see your doctor! Drop all the machismo crap, release any fears about cancer and just go! There are many other reasons you may not be *p*eeing the way you used to. Don't let your fears or the assumption of cancer *p*revent you from getting treated for what may be a benign condition.

TABLE OF CONTENTS

My journey was not alone.

I wish to thank the innumerable friends and family who were with me both physically and in spirit. This journey would not have been the same without you.

And thanks to all the health care providers I saw on my journey. I feel as though I had the best care possible every step of the way.

And deep thanks mostly to my best friend and personal nurse, who sure isn't pretty!* Even though you didn't always believe in the path I chose, you supported me.
All my love.

---

* Many years ago, I started using the phrase "You're not just another pretty face" to compliment my wife on her intelligence. Over the years, and with a touch of our odd sense of humor, it has been shortened to simply "You sure aren't pretty".

CAPE CANAVERAL, Fla.-

NASA is unsure what caused the hydrogen gas leak that prevented space shuttle Discovery from flying, but will nonetheless attempt another launch today.

[By Marcia Dunn; AP Aerospace Writer]

The above paragraph is the beginning of an article printed in the Albuquerque Journal on March 15th, 2009. I was not yet one month out of my prostate surgery and this spoke loudly enough to me to know that I had to write this book.

What does the space shuttle Discovery have to do with prostate cancer/surgery? Well, nothing and everything. To me it speaks about the level of risk we are individually prepared to take when faced with adversity in our lives. Not foolish or careless risks, but educated, well calculated risks.

Personally, I'm not ready to risk going up in a space shuttle when they don't know what caused a previous hydrogen gas leak. But then I'm not an astronaut. Perhaps these astronauts wouldn't be ready to risk waiting 16 months after a diagnosis of prostate cancer to have surgery. I was.

And this is my story.

1

The Mantra

Once it became evident that I was going to undergo surgery, I developed a Mantra for myself which stated pretty clearly what my hopes were for the results of my radical prostatectomy:

Cancer Free
Drip Free
Fully Erect

This three part Mantra became my goal — making it part of my awareness at all times as I went through the preparation for the surgery.

Now the first part, "Cancer Free", was pretty much out of my control, once I had chosen a qualified surgeon. I honestly never gave the "Cancer Free" portion of the Mantra much thought as I assumed that was the main purpose of the surgery, so why wouldn't it turn out that way? Trusting, naive, delusional...? Now I'm not saying there was no chance of complications. Even with the best qualified surgeon, there's always the potential for something to go wrong. There's also never a guarantee the cancer hadn't spread to a different part of my body — even though I had gone through two bone scans to rule out that probability. I simply chose to trust in the surgeon to take care of his part of my mantra. And trust I did.

You can most assuredly surmise that being "Drip Free" was my main concern after the surgery, as it is the topic of this book. I had spoken with several men (and had read about more in print and online) who had gone through having a radical prostatectomy as a result of their prostate cancer, and they all had their stories regarding varying degrees of "dryness" post-surgery. Many would proclaim the surgery a complete success with no complaints until I queried them further about incontinence. This was often followed with descriptions of "a little leaking at the end of the day", or "when I strain" or something of the like. Most didn't seem concerned with this. Some were still wearing pads months or years after surgery, and some said the few drops were simply caught in their underwear. This last part I can almost understand. After all, who hasn't heard the saying "No matter how you shake and dance, the lasts few drops always go in your pants" when referring to men peeing. So, a few drops wouldn't be much more of an issue over what we men all deal with on a daily basis. It's when I heard stories of men functioning ok, but still wearing pads when they go work out at the gym, or something of the like, that got me so obsessed with stopping the post-surgical leakage!

That may be fine for them, but what about those of us who go commando and haven't worn underwear for countless years? It's enough of a lifestyle change just to be wearing underwear, but then to knowingly be dripping in them or wearing pads? No thanks! I had to do whatever it took to prevent that in the long term for my "Drip Free" quality of life.

Part 3 of the Mantra, "Fully Erect", was also not much of a concern. Now I'm not saying I don't enjoy my erections as much as the next guy, but I don't have erections nearly as often as I need to pee, so dripping vs. being flaccid seemed much more of a negative impact on one's lifestyle. Besides, this also is mostly in the hands of the surgeon, depending on (among other things) the success of nerve sparing during the operation. Also, there are several prescription drug choices for erectile dysfunction if necessary. Not to mention implants, and other devices if one chooses to go that direction.

But there's no magic pill to take that stops you from dripping! I know there are a group of antispasmodic drugs such as Dicyclomine, Ditropan, Detrol and Toviaz that "in general" work to relax the muscles of the bladder to help prevent what is called urge incontinence. However, it's not my bladder that will be the cause of my incontinence following this surgery, so I doubt the effectiveness of an antispasmodic medication in this instance.

And yes, there is also a surgically implanted, manually activated sphincter available that will assist in the starting and stopping of urine flow. But I'm talking about maximum quality of life as my goal, and none of these options fit into that model for me.

2

Surgilube and Donuts

When I was discharged from the hospital following my surgery, I of course still had my Foley in place — the catheter — the lovely door prize you are sent home with. I was to continue wearing this for two weeks. Imagine — two weeks walking around with a tube up your penis and a bag of pee strapped to your leg. Well, this is definitely part of the package when you sign up for a radical prostatectomy. And honestly, for me, this was the worst part of the recovery process.

My discharge orders were pretty simple — too simple, as it turned out. In addition to instructions as to how to empty and change the collection bags, I was told to keep the catheter clean, washing it with baby shampoo whenever it needs it, and (and this is the critical step...) lubricate it with some KY if there's any sticking or friction. Sounded miserable, but easy enough.

I made it home, bag in tow, with no drama and settled in to my new home on the couch. I thought with the catheter tubing it would be much easier to sleep alone in an upright/ reclining position instead of in bed with my wife and multiple legs thrashing around and the ever present threat of our Yorkie jumping up in the middle of the night, or our Russian Wolfhound coming to the side of the bed to wake me up while stepping on... well, you get the picture. Needless to say, I was being extremely careful of all this new apparatus — coddling my fears of it being yanked out of my bladder, or some other such nightmare.

As I settled in for sleep, I proceeded to lubricate the tubing where it exited my penis with some KY personal lubricant that we happened to have at the house. That word "friction" left me wanting to take no chances. Thanks in part to pain medication (better living through chemistry) I had a relatively good night's sleep. When I awoke, I made one of what would be many trips to the bathroom to empty "the bag". Being compliant, I also washed the tubing and applied a little more lubricant. So far so good.

The day passed as I alternated my time between changing channels and changing collection bags. There is the larger bag for the long periods of inactivity, and the smaller walking bag which straps to one's leg. I tried to walk as much as I could, going on several short trips around the neighborhood each day. I soon stopped caring that I was wearing my robe or whether the tubing or bag was showing. We had lived in our neighborhood for many years and knew most of the neighbors anyway.

As the day progressed, and the evening wore on, things started getting "interesting". Interpret that as "painful". It seemed that no matter how clean I was keeping the tubing and how much KY I was applying, the tube moving in and out of my penis had become extremely uncomfortable. There was some sort of residue forming on the tubing that was a huge source of irritation and pain. Even some bleeding was happening. Trust me when I say that you don't want to see blood coming out of the end of your penis! Well, it got so bad by the end of that second night that I was literally in tears, telling my wife there was no way I could tolerate this for the remainder of the two week sentence. It felt as if the catheter were made of sandpaper. Just imaging a rolled up piece of sandpaper sliding in and out of your penis. No, it's not pretty. The bleeding and pain had me quite freaked out.

Did I tell you that my wife is a nurse, or "was" as we like to say? She is a case manager, so not in a clinical setting, but a nurse nonetheless. She got on the phone to the floor of the hospital from where I was discharged and talked to the nurse there, describing the problem. Well, somewhere in the conversation that nurse said she didn't have anything else to offer — just lubricate with sterile KY. **Sterile!** That would have been very good information to have had upon discharge. I cannot tell you how that one word changed the remainder of my post-op experience.

We checked our medical larder and didn't have any Surgilube — the brand name of a medical equivalent of home KY. She got in the car and made a run to the nearby Walgreens — certain that they would have some. Well, after striking out she moved on to the nearest hospital emergency room. (Not just a nurse, but an extremely determined nurse when on a mission!) She managed to talk to the right people and get some small sample packages of Surgilube and rushed them home to my bleeding penis. Sorry for the visual, but that's how it was!

Now, take a little time to visualize the most beautiful, peaceful place you can think of. Get a good picture of it in your mind — don't leave out any details. You're there with the woman or man of your dreams. Everything is perfect. You are at rest and all problems are either miles away or non-existent. You are completely at peace. Got it? Nice!

This has nothing to do with what's going on, I just wanted to leave you with a more pleasant visual image...

When my wife arrived from her rescue mission to the hospital, I emptied the catheter bag, thoroughly washed the tubing, and applied the sterile Surgilube. **Aaaahhhhhh......** the sandpaper tubing was gone, and the catheter irritation was never a problem for the remainder of the two week period. If my wife did nothing else during my recovery phase, she had done enough in making that hospital run that evening!

So, in closing — use only Surgilube, or some other brand of medically **sterile** KY, if you need any lubricant. And ask for several small sample packets before you are discharged. Chances are you won't need more than that.

Now on to the donuts!

While the tubing itself wasn't causing a problem any more, a fact of the male anatomy was presenting another problem. If you trace the path of the urethra from the head of the penis until it joins the bladder, there's a significant portion that lies just under the skin of the perineum. That's the area between the anus and the scrotum, as shown on the following image:

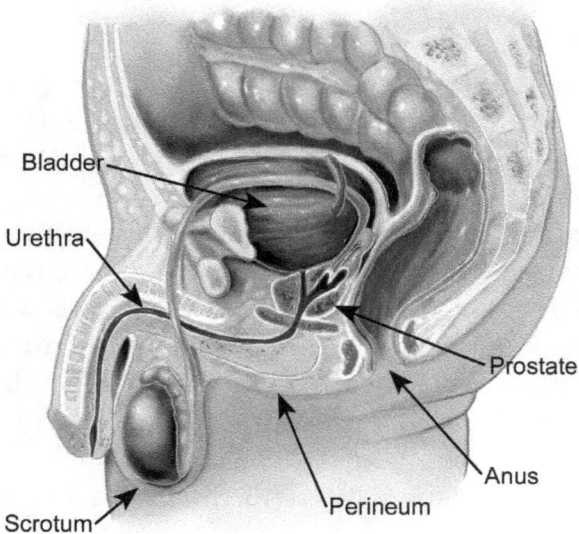

Now, normally this fact isn't much of a problem. But when there's a rather large tube running the entire length of your urethra it, of course, runs along the perineum as well. While the urethra itself is a soft, collapsible tissue, the catheter tubing is much firmer. As a result, when you sit down on a less than perfectly padded surface, the pressure of the tubing pushing against the spongy tissue of the perineum is uncomfortable and painful at times. Nothing like the sandpaper mind you, but still painful. Sorry to bring up the sandpaper again. If you have to review that serene image I had you create earlier, I'll give you some time...

Anyway, there's a very simple fix for this one. I'm assuming you've seen or at least heard about the donuts people sit on when they have hemorrhoids and such. Well, that was my original thought, and those work fine for hemorrhoids, but not a urethra being irritated from a catheter. You see, being a donut, it makes a complete circle, and a portion of that donut would still apply pressure along the urethra. Enter the neck rest to the rescue! I'm talking about the U-shaped device worn around the necks of travelers so they can take naps on planes, trains and automobiles without their head flopping around. They are just large enough so that when placed under your butt with the open portion of the u-shape facing toward the front, they protect the entire perineum area. Again, aaahhhh..... And yes, I would use it at home, in the car, and take it to restaurants and anywhere else I knew I would be sitting. Trust me — you won't care about dragging this apparatus around with you!

I know this chapter possibly should have been called "Surgilube and Neck Rests" — I just thought donuts had a nicer ring to it.

3

One sphincter, two sphincter,
Red Sphincter, blue sphincter

Time for a short anatomy lesson. And my apologies for using the word "short" in a discussion about the penis.

You see, if it was just a matter of the urethra healing up after surgery, there would be no dripping problem to speak of. What's at issue here begins with the fact that men have two urinary sphincters in their plumbing systems as opposed to the single sphincter in women. A sphincter is a muscle, or group of muscles, that clamps down around the urethra to close it off and stop the flow of urine out of the bladder. In the following figure you'll notice there's one sphincter at the base of the bladder, and another at the base of the prostate.

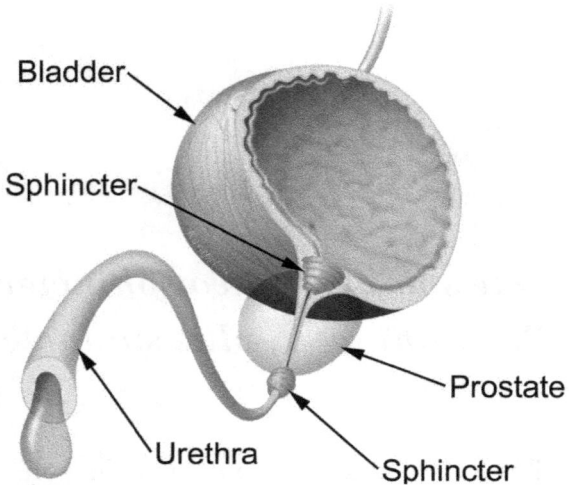

Well, when the prostate is removed, so goes the second sphincter! This is one of the problems causing dripping following surgery. Where we men are used to having a dual valve system, all of a sudden we are attempting to have the same level of control as before with only half of the equipment.

Here's my theory on the need for two sphincters in the first place, and it has to do more with sex than peeing. Let's first assume we have only one sphincter at the base of the bladder as is the case with women. Under perfect conditions, it would stay closed when we don't need or want to pee, and open when we do to allow the flow of urine from the bladder, through the urethra and out into the world. So far so good.

Now let's enter the prostate and second sphincter into the equation. You see, in addition to urine, we men have the need to allow seminal fluid to pass through the same urethra — at the appropriate time, of course. And as a man, you probably are aware that it's nearly impossible to pee when you have an erection. This is because of the dual sphincter system, and is necessary because when seminal fluid and sperm are passing through the urethra during sex, we don't want urine to be there at the same time. Urine, while being inert, is very acidic and will alter the pH of the seminal fluid which in turn will affect the viability of the sperm. Because of this, during sex the bladder sphincter will close completely, and the prostate sphincter will open at the appropriate time to allow the uninterrupted flow of sperm and seminal fluid.

This also explains the phenomenon of "morning wood". When we have to pee and are asleep, our brain often sends us an erotic dream which causes an erection, closes the sphincter at the base of the bladder, and shuts down the flow of urine. I would venture to say that an erotic dream is most always preferred over wetting the bed. Likewise, when we have an erection during sex the bladder sphincter pretty much just closes tight to prevent the seepage of urine.

At the same time, the seminal fluid still needs an egress route, and the only way is via the same urethra through which urine has previously passed. That's where the prostate sphincter comes into play. When it's "time", that sphincter opens to allow the flow of sperm and seminal fluid out the urethra, while at the same time the bladder sphincter remains closed — eliminating the flow of any urine. I believe these two sphincters are connected somehow — or at least are able to talk to one another so they remain in sync. So, when one of them is removed during surgery, the remaining sphincter is lonely and confused and thus doesn't function as well as it used to before its "twin" went missing. This is the primary reason we need to strengthen our pelvic floor muscles so they can assist and retrain your remaining sphincter.

There's not much more to say about this — it's just important information to have so you can understand why you may not have the bladder control you used to. Review the figure at the beginning of this chapter to better visualize the dual sphincter system I'm talking about.

What is important to realize is that although it may be difficult and time consuming, you can regain some, most, or all of your control again. While I have regained a vast majority of my bladder control, I don't intend to intimate that all men are the same. I totally understand this, but want you to have a good balance between despair and hope around this issue. To quote the Dalai Lama (not talking about prostate cancer, of course) " Despair is never a solution."

4

Sexercise

Finally the big day — my post-op appointment! This was the day they were to remove the catheter. Even though I had become adept at emptying and changing bags and managed to navigate the entire two week period without spilling even a drop, I cannot tell you how much I was looking forward to having this new appendage removed!

I sort of knew what to expect during this "procedure". That word makes it seem so simple and sterile, doesn't it? Yet all the while they're dealing with one of the most intimate parts of your body. At the end of the catheter, inside the bladder, is a small balloon which is inflated with saline when the catheter is first put in place. This keeps the catheter from being accidentally pulled out — yikes! So, the first step is to use a syringe to empty the proper amount of saline out of the balloon to ensure it's empty. Once that's done, it's just a matter of a simple tug and whoosh — it's out! And so it was.

Now comes the messy part. I was pretty much just handed a few paper towels, had the sink pointed out to me and told the doctor would be in soon to see me. What...? That's it...?! You must realize at this point that after having a catheter in place for two weeks you basically have no control whatsoever over the flow of urine. Waddling over to the sink, pants around my ankles, I soon realized I needed more paper towels — which, thankfully, were available. There was also a "pad" that was shown to me earlier and placed on the counter — conveniently out of reach. Why wasn't it placed near the sink?! Anyway, my wife handed the pad to me, and after managing to stop the major amounts of flow (I'm sure it was just that I was finally approaching empty) I put the pad in place in my underwear, pulled them up, and promptly proceeded dripping into the pad. Yes, for the first time since childhood I was peeing in my pants! Even knowing the pad was securely in place, it just didn't feel right.

My doctor came in, examined the scar, told me how well the surgery went (really, really well!), wished me luck and told me he would see me in 6 months.

–drip, drip, drip...--

Really? That's it? I'm done? I guess I was hoping for a little more information about the dripping that was going on in my pants. I asked someone about that and was handed a single sheet of paper describing the Kegel exercises. They may have said something like "Make sure you do these", but I really can't remember. I was still in a little bit of shock.

–drip, drip, drip...–

So, I proceeded to leave the hospital and head for the nearest medical supply store to stock up on adult diapers. I'll spare you the details here, but basically I bought a case of expensive diapers only to find out later that they were not covered by insurance...! (Don't get me started on the fact that the Erectile Dysfunction drugs are covered, but the diapers and pads are not!)

OK — back to the Kegels. And herein lies one of the worst ironies of this whole experience. About halfway down this single sheet of instructions, is the sentence:

"It is helpful to start performing Kegels 1-2 weeks prior to surgery."

What? I was supposed to start these two weeks before my surgery and I'm just reading this now?! After enduring two weeks of living with the catheter, standing in the exam room tubing free and dripping uncontrollably, continuing to drip in my pants as I purchased my first case of diapers, and I'm finally advised of this?!?

To be honest, I had heard a little something about these exercises before and had, in fact, started doing them a tiny bit prior to the surgery, but hadn't really taken them seriously. In retrospect, pre-surgical exercise certainly makes sense. It's like training for a race, versus running cold — not well advised. So, once settled in at home, I proceeded to do the Kegels quite faithfully and with a fair amount of success. But after a few months, and being a little impatient, I wanted to find out if there was more that could be done.

I happened to be seeing my chiropractor one day and mentioned my problem with incontinence that I had been experiencing since surgery — even with doing the Kegels. A light went on in his head and he suggested that I talk to this other body worker in his office who, among many other things, teaches exercises primarily for just this problem. I had seen her for other body work in the past, so before I left his office I had an appointment with her to learn about what she called "Sexercise".

In general, this is a group of exercises derived from the Pilates system that she teaches, primarily to women, to strengthen the entire pelvic floor. The name "Sexercise" is used because, while tightening up the pelvic floor muscles aids in incontinence, it also has the effect of making sex more pleasurable. Not a bad secondary gain! Since you are down to one sphincter following your prostatectomy, as described in Chapter 3, the only way to gain more urinary control is to strengthen the musculature surrounding the urethra — the pelvic floor. These exercises are like Kegels on steroids!

Step 1. Moving the sits bones together.

Your sits bones are quite literally the bones you sit on — underneath the fleshy part of your butt. (Technically, the ischial tuberosity.) See the following diagram to clarify.

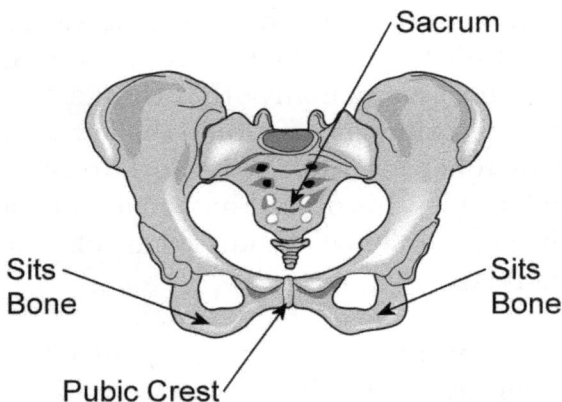

To execute this first step, lie on your back, with your knees bent, your feet flat on the floor and arms at your side. Visualize your sits bones and imagine them moving closer together. Initially, all you may be able to do is visualize, and that's ok. You might need to practice a few times just to figure out how to engage the muscles that would make them move closer together. If you can, it's helpful to reach around with your hands and feel the sits bones as you start tightening various muscles until you engage the right ones. Now, will your sits bones actually move? It doesn't matter — engaging the muscles is what's important. This is what will strengthen the pelvic floor. Hold these muscles for several seconds and release. Repeat for 8-10 repetitions, or whatever feels comfortable. Like any exercise program, start off slowly until you're sure you're doing it correctly.

Step 2. Moving the sacrum closer to the pubic crest.

This step is similar to Step 1, it just involves moving a different set of bones — the sacrum (tail bone) and the pubic crest. The sacrum is the small, triangular plate located at the base of your spine. The pubic crest (symphysis) is the hard bone you can feel at the base of your penis. Refer back to the diagram in step one if you need to review the location of the bones.

Continue lying on your back with knees up, as in Step 1. The focus here is to move the sacrum closer to the pubic crest. Again, you may not actually feel anything moving, but the goal is to strengthen the muscles that would move them. Similar to Step 1, you may wish to place your fingers on the pubic crest. You just might feel it moving down (towards the sacrum) a little bit! Hold for several second and release. Repeat for the same 8-10 repetitions as in Step 1.

Step 3. Doing step 1 and step 2 at the same time.

Once you've mastered the first two steps, it's time to combine them into one movement. The goal here is to tighten the all muscles from Step 1 and Step 2 at the same time.

You might have better luck in the beginning tightening the sits bones muscles first, then adding the sacrum/pubic crest muscles. Eventually you will be able to do this all in one movement. Hold for several seconds and release, then repeat for the appropriate number of repetitions.

Step 4. While performing Step 3, drawing all the muscles upward.

Now for the grand finale. And I do mean grand! This step is to be added once you have mastered Step 3.

Let's start with another visualization. Imagine all the muscles you've used in Step 3 above. All the muscles to move the sits bones together, and all the muscles used to move the sacrum closer to the pubic crest meet in one central point. This is the foundation of the pelvic floor, which is what you are now using to regain control of your urination.

While you have a good hold on all the muscles mentioned above (Step 3), this final step is to focus on that central point and pull that point upward, moving parallel with your spine. Picture all of the muscles forming a nice cone shape as you do this, with the base of the cone on your pelvic floor, and the tip of the cone somewhere above that. As with all the steps, hold for several second and release; repeat.

It is recommended to start doing all of these exercises lying flat as described in the beginning of Step 1. However, with time and practice, you will be able to do them anywhere and in most any position — sitting, driving, walking, even running. With enough practice, you will be able to focus only on this last Step 4 — pulling the pelvic floor upwards — and all the other muscles will react as trained. And, like Kegels, no one will know you're doing them. Although, in the beginning you will have this odd look of concentration on your face that will keep people guessing!

5

A bicycle built for who...?

After a month or so of Sexercise (see Chapter 4) I was extremely pleased with the level of bladder control I was experiencing. Then came our 25th wedding anniversary. Seemingly unrelated, I know — bear with me while I explain.

I planned a surprise trip to San Francisco for my wife and me to celebrate together. We always loved that city and hadn't been there for a while. Among the usual things one does in San Francisco, we decided to rent bicycles one day and ride through Golden Gate Park. Since neither of us are avid, or even occasional riders, we opted for the electric-assist bikes. Won't go into details on those, but really, really nice!

The weather was quite cold and windy that day, but we had a great time nonetheless. But let me explain the whole mechanics of bicycle seats to you. Those of you who do ride bikes frequently may already know this.

Remember the "Donuts" section of Chapter 2 where I describe the path the urethra takes along the perineum? Well, that perineum rests firmly on the tip of a standard bicycle seat. That also happens to be where a lot of your weight can rest while riding. Needless to say, this causes way too much stress and irritation to that whole area, and that one day of riding managed to undo much of the hard work I had been doing with all the Sexercise. Maintaining continence for the next day or two was difficult. Fortunately, with no more bicycle riding and continued Sexercise, I was able to get back to where I was before. In retrospect however, I would definitely have skipped the whole bike excursion if I had know the consequences beforehand.

While we're talking about bicycle seats, I must mention the effect bicycle riding may have on your PSA level. The PSA blood test is far from perfect, as there are more reasons for an elevated PSA level beyond having prostate cancer. For example, as men age, it's typical for the prostate to get enlarged. While a "normal" sized prostate may put out an acceptable level of PSA, a larger prostate will put out a higher level. It's the whole bigger engine syndrome — you get more horse power out of a larger engine.

Inflammation, or swelling of the prostate (prostatitis) is also a potential reason for an elevated PSA level. An infection (prostatitis) can certainly cause inflamation, but so can some forms of external irritation such as pressure from a bicycle seat. You can actually feel your prostate if you press on the correct area of the perineum (See diagram in Chapter 2), as it's not that far below the surface of your skin. Since the perineum rides hard on a bicycle seat, an extended amount of riding can irritate and inflame your prostate, causing an elevated PSA level.

If you find your PSA level rising, and you're an avid cyclist, you may try not riding for a month or so and rechecking your PSA level. I personally know men who have tried this and their PSA level dropped significantly. There are also many kinds of "split-seats" that take the pressure off the perineum so you can keep on riding. Just know that not riding a bicycle is by no means a cure for anything! If you think you can put off getting your PSA level checked just because you've stopped riding your bike, you are sadly mistaken. Even though the PSA test has its faults, it is still something that should be followed by all men, in my opinion, who are over the age of 40 — especially if you have any family history of the disease. Remember, avoiding the test won't prevent cancer!

6

Would you like fries with that?

While meeting with one of the prospective surgeons for my operation, I inquired (somewhat jokingly) if he could perform a vasectomy "while he was in there". I fully understood that a vasectomy usually involved a small incision in the scrotum and that he was going to be busy in my lower abdomen — not even close. But I figured a question unasked is a question unanswered. Expecting maybe a little chuckle or an explanation of why that wasn't possible, I was quite surprised when he told me that a vasectomy was pretty much part of the package — everyone getting a radical prostatectomy gets a vasectomy at the same time. It's not exactly the same as the "normal" procedure, but the vas deferens gets severed nonetheless with the same resulting infertility.

Now in my case, that was fine, because I had wanted a vasectomy anyway. But what about those men who are young enough to still want to have children (technically, me included) and don't bother to ask? Mind you, with the prostate gland gone you will primarily be having dry orgasms, but if the testicles were still hooked up to the "system" I see no reason someone with no prostate couldn't still procreate. The prostate, after all, is responsible for the production of seminal fluid — not the sperm. That's the job of the testicles. Hmmm... I didn't ask about those — maybe I should take a look.

But seriously, even if procreation wouldn't be possible through normal sexual copulation following your prostatectomy, you might want the opportunity to harvest some sperm for later use. Harvesting and storing sperm (cryopreservation or freezing) is something many persons or couples do for various personal reasons. It would be nice to have a little warning to give you time for the harvesting, or at least consider the possibility.

The "procedure" for harvesting sperm

prior to surgery is a simple matter of catching the ejaculate. Granted, you can have sperm harvested (sperm aspiration) after the prostatectomy, but that involves either a needle or another surgery — on the scrotum and testicles! So why go through all that when you can simply do something before your surgery that you are most likely well practiced in already.

7

Diapers and pads and shields, oh my!

Unsure of what my level of urinary control would be right after surgery, I started out using diapers as soon as the catheter was removed. I didn't want to be leaking anywhere at anytime, so I figured regardless of how uncomfortable they may be, I'm opting for maximum protection.

Did I mention uncomfortable? Having my pelvis wrapped in plastic and being limited to only a few of my baggier pants was definitely not my cup of tea. I couldn't help but imagine, as our population continues to age, if this is what was in store for all of us. Perhaps the practice with these diapers would make me a little better prepared than some? Understandably, I was looking for a silver lining!

Soon I was able to graduate to the smaller, somewhat less uncomfortable pads that slip inside the cup of your underwear. Still not the same as going commando like I was used to, but at least most of my pelvis could breathe a little better through the cotton.

Note to men who wear boxers — there's no cup in boxers! You'll have to outfit yourselves with a new wardrobe of underwear that has a cup.

Note to those of you who (like myself) go commando — yes, any underwear with a cup will suffice. I know, it's a lot to get used to.

Note to all — whatever underwear you buy, get them a little larger than usual. You'll need room to stuff that small mattress in there.

There are numerous choices for brands and sizes of men's incontinence pads. Not the same array as the choice of menstrual or incontinence products for women, but choices nonetheless. I found that the pads gave me a relative freedom and comfort far beyond the diapers. Now, since pads only work while wearing underwear, I was still using diapers at night for a while. They were looser than the pads, and somewhat more comfortable for evening wear. Interestingly enough, from the day I had the catheter removed, I never really had any leaks to mention while sleeping. Fortunately this meant I was able to abandon the diapers completely within the first month.

Working dutifully on the Kegels (had yet to discover Sexercise) I was drying up pretty well and was ready to "downsize" my pads. For the relatively tiny amount I was leaking, the pads seemed like so much overkill. Silly me — I thought it would be as simple as going to the store and picking up a box of thin pads — the next step. Well, guess what? There weren't any!

Several people — my wife included — suggested that I try some of the feminine "light days" products, since they are much thinner than the incontinence pads that are generally sold for men. Now, it's emasculating enough to be buying incontinence products at all, much less waltzing down the feminine hygiene aisle of the supermarket and picking up a pretty pink package of "panty liners", or other such product. But besides the embarrassment factor, allow me to explain a bit anatomically why those really wouldn't work. If you notice the shape of a women's protective shield, it's a narrow strip of absorbent material. Compare that with the shape externally of a vagina — pretty similar. Also, the vagina doesn't move around — it tends to stay in the same place from hour to hour, day to day. So, if a protective shield is placed in front of it, you can be relatively assured it's going to catch whatever is dripping out. Especially if it has wings!

Let's contrast that to a man's "package". The testicles are doing the best they can to maintain their core temperature to ensure the health and safety of your "boys". The sac will tighten and loosen throughout the day to help regulate that temperature, so you already have some movement going on there.

Now let's talk about the penis. Yes, it does seem to have a mind of its own. And whereas a vagina stays in place, the penis is continually growing and shrinking and generally flopping around all the time. To quote Elaine Benes from Seinfeld while talking to George and Jerry about "shrinkage": *"I don't know how you guys walk around with those things."* So you see, if the penis happened to be in the right place at the right time, a women's thin menstrual strip would work great. This was something I just wasn't wanting to leave to chance. What I wanted was a thin pad that covered all possible flopping areas, and I wasn't having any luck finding them.

Enter Google® to the rescue! I won't go into detail, but here's what I found:

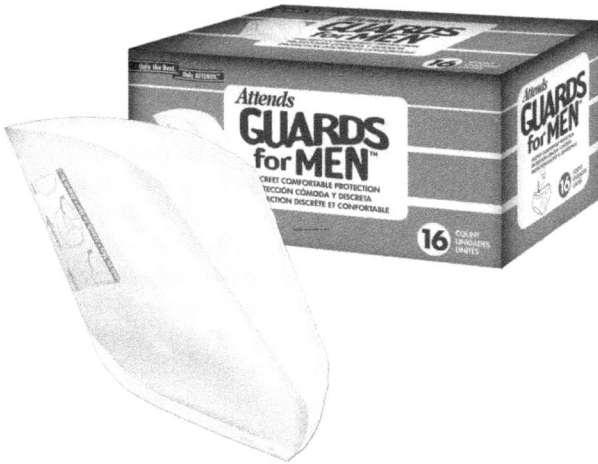

These can be purchased at:

http://www.justattends.com

or

1-800-322-2721

This product is a nice, thin, absorbent cup which fits inside your underwear, with an adhesive strip on the outside to hold it in place. It comfortably surrounds the entire area of potential leakage. They won't handle a flood, but when you are finally down to just some minor leakage and want to have a little protection when you go out, these fit that need perfectly.

There is one small caveat to using these. On the inside bottom of the cup is a seam from the manufacturing of the product. If you wear them "out-of-the-box" that seam will separate enough to expose a small strip of adhesive that insists on sticking to your scrotum. Not the most pleasant of experiences! A couple of appropriately placed pieces of scotch tape will prevent that from happening.

Let me just say that I now have a much greater appreciation for the plethora of choices down the "feminine hygiene" aisles in stores. As with women, all men are not the same and we like to have choice (and comfort) as well. So, if you don't like the product(s) you're using, take some time to dig around a little. The Attends® product mentioned earlier in this chapter may not be for you, but you should be able to find something that is.

8

My Timeline

I thought I would share with you the chronological course of events leading up to and following my prostatectomy. It started probably sometime in 1998 when I first noticed a reduction in my urine stream — I couldn't pee with as much force as I used to. My doctor first thought it may just be an enlarged prostate and put me on the drug Flomax® for a couple of weeks to see if it made a difference. It didn't. The next step was to start checking my PSA level.

And so it began:

February 2, 1999   PSA 2.3

September 27, 2001   PSA 3.7

February 12, 2002   PSA 3.2

June 9, 2003   PSA 3.4

January 8, 2004   PSA 3.7

November 3, 2005   PSA 4.2

December 19, 2005   Needle biopsy

12 biopsies; 6 from the left, 6 from the right

Pathology report:

Diagnosis: Without diagnostic abnormality.
i.e. negative: no evidence of cancer

July 18, 2006   PSA 4.9

October 3, 2007   PSA 6.36

October 21, 2007   Ran a marathon

November 8, 2007   Needle biopsy

12 biopsies; 6 from the left, 6 from the right

Pathology report:

Diagnosis A: Right Prostate.
Adenocarcinoma of the prostate, Gleason grade

3+3 (Score 6/10) involving approximately 5% of the specimen (tumor is present in one of six cores). Focal high grade prostatic intraepithelial neoplasia.

i.e. positive: cancer

Diagnosis B: Left Prostate. Focal high grade prostatic intraepithelial neoplasia. Glandular hyperplasia and patch acute/ chronic inflammation.

December 28, 2007   PSA 6.65

January 11, 2008
Nuclear medicine whole body bone scan
Impression: No convincing evidence of metastatic disease.

January 29, 2008   PSA 7.53

March 5, 2008   MRI -
                         Prostate gland

Findings:

The prostate gland is mildly enlarged. There is abnormal low signal involving the peripheral and central zones of the prostate gland on the right. The patient has biopsy proven adenocarcinoma involving the right lateral aspect of the prostate gland.

Prostate gland does not extend into the surrounding soft tissues. The facial and fat planes are preserved surrounding the prostate gland.

Impression:

Mild enlargement of the prostate gland.

Abnormal low signal within the peripheral and central zones of the prostate gland on the right compatible with the patient's known carcinoma in this location.

March 21, 2008   PSA 8.74

April 25, 2008   PSA 9.59

June 12, 2008   PSA 8.30

September 22, 2008   PSA 10.00

January 20, 2009   PSA 14.00

February 18, 2009   Surgery

Radical Prostatectomy

Pathology report:

Diagnosis:
Prostatic Adenocarcinoma, Gleason's 4+4=sum 8 of 9 total points (poorly differentiated prostatic adenocarcinoma).

Tumor is confined to the right side of the prostate extending posteriorly to anteriorly.

Margins of resection negative for tumor with tumor closely approaching the right anterior portion of the prostate for a distance of 5mm (tumor is located approximately 0.1mm (0.01cm) from the inked tissue edge).

Tumor does not involve seminal vesicles, apex, base, opposite side of prostate, extraprostatic tissue, or prostatic urethra.

Negative for lymphovascular invasion.

Additional findings of chronic cystitis of the prostatic urethra, benign prostatic hyperplasia, and focal nonspecific chronic prostatitis.

Tumor is staged as: T2B/NX/MX by AJCC Cancer Staging Manual, 6th Edition.

March 3, 2009
Post-op appointment.

CATHETER REMOVED! (See Chapter 4)

March 15, 2009
Went running for the first time post-surgery.
Had a pad in my shorts, but stayed dry!

October 12, 2009   PSA 0.07

February 4, 2010   PSA 0.08

September 6, 2010   PSA 0.10

I will continue to monitor my PSA level at whatever frequency my doctor recommends.

So, just where am I in my quest to be "drip free"? Pretty damn close, I'd say. For one thing, diapers, pads and shields are totally a thing of the past. All told, I think I went through about a dozen diapers, maybe 2 packages of pads (12 to a package) and one box of 64 of the Attends shields. Today I am back to full commando, with very few exceptions. If I'm going somewhere a little more formal and am wearing some light pants, I may put on a pair of underwear — just in case. Or if I've had a really long day and am physically tired, I may need to go to the bathroom more frequently. And that's just about it.

Well, then there's farting. (Do I even want to go there?) The practice of farting is related to the sphincters talked about in Chapter 3. You see, besides the bladder and prostate sphincters, there's another sphincter in the neighborhood — the anal sphincter. That's what opens to let out, among other things, a good fart. But picture this: you are having some trouble peeing so you're standing there at the urinal when you decide to push out what you can. Often when you do this, you inevitably let out a fart in the process. There seems to be a connection (the pelvic floor?) between the bladder sphincter and the anal sphincter as well. So, if pushing out some pee results in a fart leaking out, the converse will also be true. That is, pushing out a fart will result in some pee leaking out. Do you really want to push out a fart when you're already having at least some trouble holding in pee? There is a fix. With proper practice of the Sexercise in Chapter 4, you will be able to keep those core pelvic floor muscles tight while at the same time "allowing" a fart to happen. You cannot push it out, but you can relax the door and let it find it's own way out.

9

Some personal thoughts on cancer

I know this book is about all the urinary issues I experienced following a radical prostatectomy, but I also wanted to include some of my thoughts and observations when I had cancer, and on cancer in general.

The day was December 27, 1987. I had just finished riding up the chair lift at Sandia Ski Area in Albuquerque with a friend. "Let's go this way" I said when we got off the lift. And that was pretty much the last thing I would remember for the next several weeks or so. You see, I was unknowingly on my way to a collision course with a tree. And, in the world of sports injuries, a human head versus a solid tree usually doesn't have a very good outcome. I was pretty fortunate — a little bleeding (ok — a lot of bleeding), some relatively minor brain damage, and some loss of motor skills, but I survived. I wouldn't say that I had a near death experience, but I can certainly say that I did come close to getting killed that day. This left me with a radically different outlook on life in general. I don't take things as seriously as before — no need for the drama. This certainly applied to getting the news that I had prostate cancer.

I also give credit to my study of the "Now". Whether it's Dan Millman's "Way of the Peaceful Warrior" or Ekhart Tolle's "The Power of Now", it's really all about living in the moment. Even Cesar Millan, the dog whisperer says dogs live only in the now. And at that moment of diagnosis, there was only cancer; no prognosis, no treatments, no surgery, certainly no death sentence, and comfortably no fear.

One could also go the direction of Zen Buddhism. The last line of "Text of the Hsin Hsin Ming Verses on the Faith Mind" by Sosan Zenji, Third Zen Patriarch states:

The Way is beyond language, for in it there is

> *no yesterday*
> *no tomorrow*
> *no today*

Also prevalent in the study of Buddhism is the concept of duality. There is no "cancer" and "no cancer". They are one and the same.

That's going in a bit of a different direction, but you get my point.

I can remember very clearly the day I was told I had cancer. I had called my urologist earlier in the day to see if the results of the biopsy were in. My wife and I were driving up North to Santa Fe for the day with our foreign exchange student from Brasil to visit a Tibetan Buddhist temple. We were just a few minutes from the parking area for the temple when he called back on my cell. "The test came back positive" he said, or something of the like. He went on into a little detail about the percentages of malignant cells in the samples and such. Medical jargon that my wife, being a nurse, would have understood more than I. "So, it's cancer?" I had to query him. He answered back in the affirmative. But it wasn't until I used the word, that he himself actually and finally said "cancer".

What is it about this word that people seem to be afraid of, I started to think? I didn't realize it until after I was diagnosed, that many people have an aversion to even saying it. There were friends and relatives that would simply ask how I was doing, interspersed with several pregnant pauses. Others would ask how my "condition" was. "Oh, you mean the cancer?" I would sometimes ask back. Not wanting to be glib about it, just calling it by name. It was quite a surprise for me to discover a general fear of cancer in our society. People will participate in all sorts of reckless behaviors and call them by name. "I'm trying to quit smoking." "I really should lose some weight — my cholesterol is up." "I'm going hang gliding this weekend." "I got another speeding ticket yesterday." Any or all of these behaviors could, but don't necessarily, lead to death. It's the same with cancer, so why can't we say "I have cancer?".

Now, I'm not exactly recommending experiencing a head injury to change your view of cancer, or the world at large, but I would like to suggest releasing your fear of cancer. "It's just cancer", after all!

In no way am I intending to discount the potential that cancer has. I have friends and relatives who have had cancer; some have even died from it. As I finish writing and editing this book, I just received a call with news that a longtime friend who was diagnosed with stage 4 pancreatic cancer only four months ago, has just died. I also worked as a volunteer on the pediatric oncology floor of a major cancer hospital for four years. So you see, I know what cancer can do to a person, and those around him/her. And, if I should someday die from cancer, it will still be "just cancer" to me.

This is not to say I wasn't surprised to hear that I had cancer. There was no history of prostate or any other form of cancer in my family. And I was healthy. I had just finished running my first marathon at age 50 in 4 hours and 4 minutes after months of training. I was in great shape. I had a healthy diet. So, there was no "reason" for me to develop cancer. Cancer, apparently, doesn't need a reason.

So, off I went on my journey to rid my body of this inconvenient invasion. Early in my research of possible treatments, I was finding one thing in common. There was a high likelihood of some degree of incontinence following either surgery or radiation — the two primary paths men choose. As I stated in the first chapter about my Mantra, this seemed like too much of a lifestyle change for me. I had to find some other way of dealing with this.

This path I chose is exactly why it took 16 months after diagnosis for me to agree to surgery. I was determined to find an alternative way to cure myself of cancer and thus avoid the conventional treatments, and side effects, altogether. I dove deep into the world of alternative or complimentary therapies with my whole heart and soul. Weeks and months passed as I researched and tried whatever treatments I could. I was also blessed with a fantastic therapist who guided me along many steps of the way. And a urologist that was open enough to let me try things on my own time, while still following my progress and monitoring my PSA level. I will not mention the numerous treatments I received, as this isn't a book about alternative therapies for cancer. Suffice it to say it was exhausting and very expensive as these types of treatments and therapies generally aren't covered by insurance.

Obviously, these treatments didn't have the effect I desired, as I watched my PSA rise over time until finally that second biopsy tested positive for cancer. Do I have any regrets for following that path and giving myself all that time to make the final decision about surgery? Not really a regret as much as an unfortunate consequence of my actions. You see, I dove into my treatments so completely, I let my body go physically. If you remember, I was diagnosed a scant two weeks after finishing my first marathon, so I was in really good shape. Today I find myself on the seeming slow road to regaining that body I had before. But even as I look at my skinny arms and legs and much larger stomach than I used to have in the mirror, it was still worth it to wait those 16 months. You see, that was the risk I was willing to take.

I fully believe that all the alternative and integrative therapies got me really clean and strong internally. I have no doubt this greatly helped my recovery. In fact, compared to the urinary inconvenience, recovering from the surgery itself was quite easy.

As I finish this book, I am currently reading all the Harry Potter books for the first time — just about half way through "The Half Blood Prince" right now, to be exact. I was surprised to find inspiration from Albus Dumbledore in Book 1 — "Harry Potter and the Sorcerer's Stone". Throughout this and all the books, most everyone uses the phrases "You-Know-Who" or "He-Who-Must-Not-be-Named" when talking about the dark lord

Voldemort. Well, in a conversation with Harry Potter about Voldemort, Professor Dumbledore says to Harry:

> *"Call him Voldemort, Harry. Always use the proper name for things. Fear of a name increases fear of the thing itself."*

Thank you Albus!

In Conclusion:

Everyone has a story, and this is mine. I hope you've found something useful in these pages for this shared journey of ours. I'm sorry you had to join me.

While I feel I had an excellent surgeon and excellent care all the way around, there was just one thing that seemed to be missing from the whole experience. The information I've shared with you here was severely lacking in my medical education prior to and following the surgery. It would have made a huge difference in my recovery and subsequent quality of life and I hope it has found its way to you in time to make a difference in yours.

You now have your own story and I'm grateful you've chosen to take me along for part of it. Continued health to you!

OK — I gotta go *pee!*

For information on ordering this book
and links to other resources
please visit the website at:

http://www.drip-free.com